Understanding

CARING

C000319096

Carers National Association

Published by Family Doctor Publications Limited
in association with the British Medical Association

Family Doctor Publications, 10 Butchers Row, Banbury, Oxon OX16 8JH

Medical Editor: Dr Tony Smith
Consultant Editors: Gail Elkington, Jill Harrison, Sue Thomas,
                        Maria Stasiak and Chris McLaughlin
Cover Artist: Dave Eastbury
Illustrator: Angela Christie
Design: MPG Design, Blandford Forum, Dorset
Printing: Reflex Litho, Thetford, Norfolk, using acid-free paper

ISBN: 1-898205-44-2

Contents

Introduction

There are estimated to be almost six million carers in Britain, people who are looking after a sick or disabled relative or friend. One in ten carers spends more than 50 hours a week caring, in some cases for many years. Most carers are between the ages of 45 and 64, although many are younger people (including children) or over pensionable age. This book is aimed primarily at a fit adult looking after another sick and/or elderly adult, although a lot of the information will be relevant to people in other situations.

Becoming a carer is usually something that starts as a result of circumstances, rather than a position you apply for as such! It might be that the person you are caring for has had an accident and suddenly you are a carer. Alternatively, you may take on the role gradually, perhaps because the person has a progressive illness such as Alzheimer's disease, and they are becoming increasingly confused and less able to manage without help. You may not even like them very much, but decide to care for them anyway because of pressure or circumstances. We have used the term 'relative' throughout this book to refer to the person you are caring for, although of course some people will be caring for a person to whom they are not related.

Many people find caring both tiring and stressful and don't know about the support and welfare benefits that may be available. If you are someone who is reluctant to seek help, do remember that you are doing an important and valuable job as a carer and, although no one is offering to pay you the going rate, you should take up such benefits that are available to help you to do your job well.

The first six chapters give practical advice on the day-to-day business of looking after someone as a carer, and also highlights the importance of looking after yourself. The next three chapters deal in detail with what support is available and how to get it – services of all kinds, financial and practical assistance, and where to turn for specific kinds of help and back-up. Finally, the appendix of useful addresses contains contact details for the many organisations and agencies which can offer specific advice and information on every aspect of life as a carer. All the organisations mentioned in the text are listed there.

KEY POINTS

✓ There are estimated to be almost six million carers in Britain

✓ One in ten carers spends more than 50 hours a week caring

✓ Caring is time consuming, tiring and stressful so you should take advantage of any assistance available

Personal care

Good personal care is of vital importance, both to maintain the morale of the person you are caring for, and to prevent minor health problems developing into more serious ones.

BATHING

A daily bath or shower is essential to maintain cleanliness and prevent odours which can develop quickly if a person is immobile. This is an area in which safety is of vital

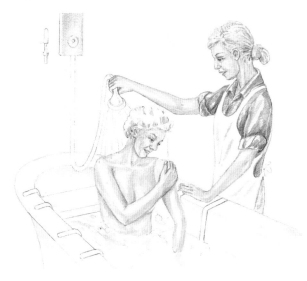

If possible, a daily bath or shower maintains cleanliness.

ESSENTIALS FOR BATHING

- A non-slip rubber bath mat (available from chemists) is advisable, although these are not suitable for some modern fibreglass baths.
- Stick adhesive shapes with anti-slip surfaces to the bottom of the bath.
- Side rails on baths are sometimes useful but do not always provide sufficient leverage. It may be necessary to fit a rail across the bath and secure it to the taps.
- Bath seats can make it easier to get in and out of the bath.
- If your relative prefers to bathe alone, make sure that the bathroom door is not locked and you are within earshot.
- Drain the bath of water before getting the person out. If the water is left in the bath it will act as a suction holding the bather in the bath.
- Installing a scald-proof temperature control on the water heater is a useful precaution.

importance; your local occupational therapist, district nurse or the Disabled Living Foundation may be able to suggest useful pieces of equipment to make bathing easier and safer. Before you start to give someone a bath or shower, make sure that you will be able to accomplish the task and that help is available if needed.

Do not use soap if the skin is irritated; alternatively switch to non-irritating soap. Change the water whenever necessary (and also if it cools down). Wear disposable plastic gloves when you wash an incontinent person for your hygiene and safety, because of intestinal bacteria. Dry the skin well, especially in the folds of the skin (groins, armpits, between the buttocks and between the toes). This will prevent irritation and soreness developing. Some patients enjoy washing their own hands and face, and may want to wash their hands actually in a bowl of water. This can be balanced on the bed. Allowing the person to wash around their own groin, if able, maintains dignity.

If bathing is too difficult showers are a good alternative but can be expensive to fit. A much cheaper alternative is to buy one of the rubber sprays which can be fitted over existing bath taps and make an effective substitute for a proper shower. Someone who is unsteady would be better sitting on a bath board rather than standing to have a shower.

After washing be sure to rinse well and dry the skin thoroughly, especially between fingers and toes. Pay attention to the underarm area and folds in the breast or groin region. Baby lotion or oil will keep the skin supple and prevent it becoming dry and flaky. A bedbath

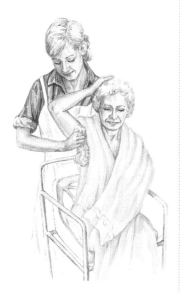

After washing, dry skin thoroughly.

is a refreshing alternative if a bath or shower is difficult.

EAR CARE

Before performing any task like this be sure to wash your own hands properly. Wash ears daily in warm water and rinse well before drying thoroughly. Do not use cotton buds to clean the inner part of the ear, as it is easily damaged. Consult your GP if wax is a problem.

EYE CARE

Using a small wad of cotton wool soaked in warm water which has previously been boiled, cleanse the eyes from the nose to the outer edge. Use a separate piece of cotton wool for each eye. This will clear the eyes of 'sleep' that accumulates overnight and prevent soreness.

HAIR CARE

If hair washing is difficult using a sink or you cannot do it in the bath or shower, there are aids that will help. You may find it easier if your relative has the bowl of water on the knees and bends the head forward.

Alternatively, you can buy a hair washing bowl to use in bed. You and your relative may prefer to have a mobile hairdresser who will come to your home and women especially often find having their hair done a good morale booster.

Washing can be tiresome and painful for someone who is frail and ill. Ensure that you discuss bedbathing with the person you care for and decide on when he or she feels up to it and what time of day is best. Also find out what he or she wants to wash alone. For someone who has to spend long periods of time in bed, washing that person's hands and face regularly is very refreshing. To wash someone in bed, you need:

- A bowl of warm water
- Towels and flannels
- Soap.

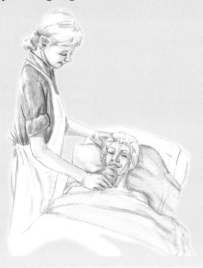

Make sure that you will not be disturbed and that the room is warm and draft free. Place a towel beneath the person you are going to bedbath.

Help with undressing and leave him or her covered with a top sheet for warmth. Wash and dry every part of the body in turn (first the face, then the chest, etc.). Keep to the following routine:

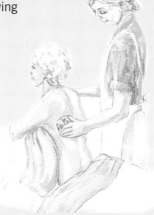

- Face
- Chest
- Arms
- Back.

Then you may wish to dress the upper part of the body to ensure warmth and dignity.

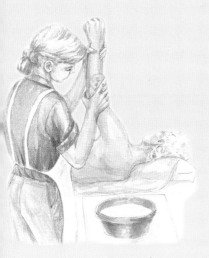

- Legs
- Lower body and groin.

Change the water.

You can then roll the person on to their side to wash:

- Lower back
- Behind the legs
- Buttocks.

Mouth care

Teeth should be brushed carefully so as to avoid gum damage. An electric toothbrush is an easy way of maintaining independence in mouth care. Some dentists make domiciliary visits if your relative can't get to the surgery. Contact the British Society of Dentistry for details of your nearest dentist with an interest in people with a disability. Mouth washes are refreshing and help to keep the mouth clean but are not a substitute for teeth cleaning. If the lips tend to become dry or chapped, try applying lip salve.

It is important to care well for dentures. If they do not fit properly eating and speaking clearly may become difficult. Dentures should never be cleaned with toothpaste, which is too rough. You can buy special denture pastes, although cleaning with a nail brush and ordinary soap is just as effective. While dentures are out the mouth can be rinsed and gums gently massaged with a soft toothbrush to remove any debris. Food particles trapped under dentures may cause ulceration and discomfort. Check regularly with the dentist that dentures continue to fit well. Weight loss may alter the fit and mean your relative is likely to experience friction and a sore mouth.

Nail care

Toe and finger nails need to be kept short to prevent skin damage from

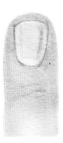

Finger nails should be kept short and rounded with rough edges smoothed away

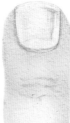

Toe nails should be cut straight across

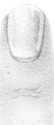

Over long nails cause injury

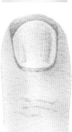

Don't cut nails too short and down at the sides

scratching. Toe nails should be cut straight across and finger nails rounded with the rough edges smoothed away. If your relative has problems with ingrown toe nails, or you are having problems cutting his or her toe nails, then he or she will need to see a chiropodist. Ask your GP for a referral. Anyone with diabetes needs thorough and careful foot care, and must also see a chiropodist regularly. Socks need to be changed daily. Avoid powdering the feet as powder can accumulate between the toes causing sweating and infection.

SHAVING

Electric razors are easier to use than the traditional wet razor if your relative has poor vision or an unsteady hand.

DISPOSAL OF WASTE

You should always wear disposable latex gloves when you are dealing

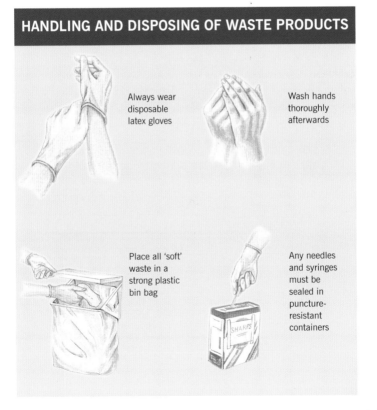

HANDLING AND DISPOSING OF WASTE PRODUCTS

Always wear disposable latex gloves

Wash hands thoroughly afterwards

Place all 'soft' waste in a strong plastic bin bag

Any needles and syringes must be sealed in puncture-resistant containers

It is extremely important to make sure your relative is comfortable, both for the sake of their general feeling of well-being and to prevent complications. Particularly:

- Ensure the bottom sheet has no wrinkles or crumbs.

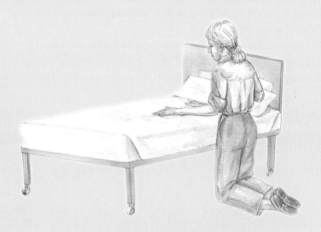

- Bed clothes should be loose enough to allow movement – duvets are preferable to blankets.

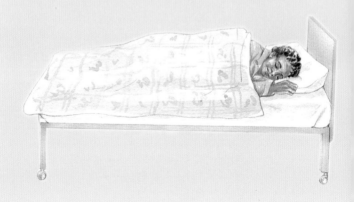

- Pillows should be positioned to give support to the back when your relative is sitting up.

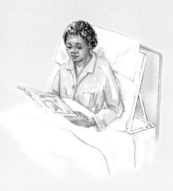

- Special pressure-relieving mattresses and beds can be obtained although they are expensive. Ask your district nurse or local Disabled Living Foundation centre about foam, gel or air cushions.

- Pillows may be positioned to prevent friction and relieve pressure.

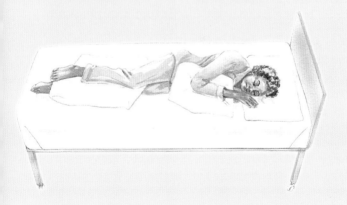

- Remember that you have to be extra careful when making the bed, if your relative is using a special mattress such as a low air loss mattress, so that you don't impede its working.

with a person's body fluids such as blood, urine, vomit or faeces. You can get gloves from the district nurse or the chemist. Gloves should also be worn if you are dressing open wounds or giving an injection. A disposal service for soiled incontinence pads is usually run by the health authority or local authority (check with social services).

Dispose of faeces down the toilet. Place soiled gloves, wipes, pads and the like in a plastic bin bag (you can get ones that are scented with a deodorant) and dispose of them in the dustbin. Always wash your hands after doing any task like this. If you have needles and syringes to dispose of seal them in puncture-resistant tins or special 'sharps' boxes – ask your district nurse for advice.

DRESSING

Do not rush dressing. If one side of the body is weaker than the other it is usually easier to begin putting clothes on this side first. When undressing take clothes off the stronger side first. Clothing can be adapted to make dressing and undressing as easy as possible. Zips and Velcro are easier to manage than buttons for people with limited coordination or manual dexterity. Socks should fit well and not bunch up under the toes, where they could cause pressure problems.

Avoid elasticated tops which can restrict the circulation or make feet swell. Tights may be difficult to get in and out of and many women prefer stockings or pop sox. It is important that shoes support the feet well. It would be best for your relative not to wear slippers all the time as they can allow the feet to swell. Techniques for dressing and adapting clothing, and aids for dressing and fastening, are discussed in the Disabled Living Foundation's excellent booklet *All Dressed Up: A Guide to Choosing Clothes and Useful Dressing Techniques for Elderly People and People with Disabilities.* They also produce a range of other useful factsheets on clothing and footwear.

EATING AND DRINKING

It is important for everyone's physical and mental well-being to eat a nutritionally balanced diet. Nutritional requirements vary according to age, activity and health. In general a healthy diet should contain reasonable amounts of protein, fibre, minerals and vitamins but not too much sugar or animal fat. Whole grains, cereals, fresh fruit and vegetables are high in vitamins and fibre, and so should be eaten as often as possible. Fibre is especially important in helping to prevent constipation in someone who is immobile. If you are concerned about your relative's diet, your district nurse or GP can advise you or refer you to a dietitian for more specific help.

If the person you care for has a poor appetite it may help to serve small meals which are light and nutritious and attractively presented. Allow plenty of time to eat meals and serve them in comfortable, quiet surroundings. Remember, if your relative spends a great deal of time in bed they may not have a big appetite. In any case it isn't easy to eat lying down, so it may help if they can have their meals sitting at a table. If your relative has difficulty getting food to their mouth, you may need to help them, or you can buy specially adapted crockery and cutlery (an occupational therapist will be able to advise you on this). When you are helping someone to eat, sit beside them and offer small mouthfuls, allowing plenty of time for chewing and swallowing before offering a further mouthful. Consider ways of keeping food hot (like stay-warm plates) if time is needed to finish a meal.

Confused people sometimes lose concentration when eating so it may be advisable to sit with them and prompt them to eat. If chewing is difficult, reducing the size of mouthfuls and providing a drink with meals can help. A speech therapist will be able to give advice on chewing and swallowing difficulties. Check also that dentures are well-fitting and in place at mealtimes. If necessary mash or liquidise food. If your relative is eating only a small range of foods you may want to consider vitamin supplements.

COMMUNICATION

Communicating effectively with the person you care for is vitally important. Difficulties in this area can be very frustrating for both of you. Imagine how you would feel if you were confined to bed and couldn't tell someone you needed to use the toilet. The problems may not relate simply to hearing and speaking; communicating is really about keeping in touch and being understood. Body language, including touch, expression, holding hands and so on, is also an important part of communication and can signify a great deal, as well as making your relative feel wanted and secure.

When you speak try to do so slowly and clearly. Ask questions you know your relative will be able to answer, even if only by shaking or nodding their head. Give the person plenty of time to respond. Some people may have difficulty because they are blind or have a particular disease or disorder, and you need to be aware of this. For example, someone with Parkinson's disease may need time to start speaking; not answering you immediately may be because they are thinking about what to say and trying to form the words. If you misunderstand their silence and carry on speaking yourself, they may lose their opportunity to communicate with you. People with dementia may use the wrong words to express something simply because they are the only words they can find. Try to interpret what you feel the person is saying more than the words you hear if this is the case. Be aware that in some cases you may hear 'mixed messages'. Be aware too that your relative may respond with verbal abuse, probably because of frustration or because the wrong words come out. Try not to let this bother you.

Sometimes there may be practical help that will improve communication. Difficulties after a stroke may be helped by a speech therapist. Difficulties in hearing may be helped by a hearing aid, although they are not always the answer; someone who is confused or who has arthritis, for example, may find one difficult to use, and it can take months of practice to get used to a new hearing aid. Your GP can refer your relative to an NHS hearing aid clinic, where a doctor will assess them, fit a suitable aid and teach them how to use it. Hearing aids are also available privately, but they may be expensive and you should get advice from your NHS clinic first. Other aids are also available, such as stereo listeners for radio or television. The Royal National Institute for Deaf People can give you more advice (see page 78).

KEY POINTS

✓ Good personal care is of vital importance to maintain morale and prevent health problems

✓ A daily bath or shower is essential for your relative

✓ Always wear disposable latex gloves when dealing with body fluids

✓ Clothing can be adapted to simplify dressing

✓ It is important for everyone to eat a nutritionally balanced diet

Inside and outside the home

ORGANISING YOUR HOME

When you become a carer, or as your caring role develops, it is worth spending some time ensuring that your home is as safe, pleasant and convenient, for both you and for the person for whom you are caring. All homes are potentially dangerous places, so safety is of vital importance.

SAFETY PRECAUTIONS

- If you must keep loose rugs, secure them with double-faced tape.
- Keep electrical flexes out of the way and where possible use cordless equipment.
- Gas appliances may need safety switches fitting, particularly if the person is confused.
- Bright lights can help prevent falls.
- Cover or pad sharp edges on furniture.
- Review kitchen and fire safety procedures. Never leave pans on the cooker if you are called away suddenly and install smoke detectors for additional safety.
- Check that stairways and hallways are properly lit. Consider installing extra handrails on stairs and in hallways.
- Furniture should be arranged to make it as easy as possible to move around the house.

- Try to make the room look as cheerful as possible – plants and flowers help brighten up the surroundings.

- The bed should be accessible from three sides to make moving and handling easier.

- The bed needs to be at an appropriate height for moving and handling. Low double beds are the worst for straining backs; single, height-adjustable ones are ideal. Your occupational therapist or district nurse is the best person to consult.

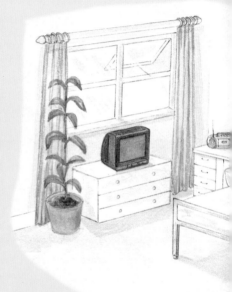

- Your relative might like a comfortable chair for when they are out of bed and another one for visitors.

- They will want a bedside table and light.

- If the bedroom isn't convenient for the toilet, you may need to get a commode which can be screened off if possible to give some privacy.

- Someone who has to spend a lot of time in their bedroom will probably like to have their own TV, radio and/or music system if possible, plus somewhere to keep books and magazines.

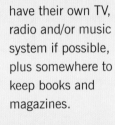

- Ensure that the room is well ventilated to allow odours to escape. Perfumed candles or air freshener are useful.

- Make sure your relative can call you if they need you – give them a bell, baby intercom or buzzer switch to ensure accessibility if you can't be certain of hearing them call.

The room your relative spends most of their time in should be comfortable, warm and well ventilated. Someone who spends all or most of their time in bed might prefer a room near the bathroom or toilet. If they need constant attention, running up and down stairs can be tiring as well as potentially hazardous for you, and you may consider moving them downstairs. On the other hand, there may be disadvantages to this, such as lack of privacy for you both, or lack of alternative toilet or bathroom facilities. When arranging your relative's room, bear the items in the box on pages 16–17 in mind.

If you do not live with the person you are caring for, then consider their security. Have a duplicate key cut; don't leave a key hanging on a string behind the letter box where anyone could get hold of it. As an additional precaution, it's worth installing door intercom and release mechanisms (your housing department or occupational therapist can give you more information). If the person you care for is confused, you may also have to fit window locks and take extra precautions to prevent unwanted callers getting in. A telephone and perhaps some other means of raising an alarm are important if the person is alone. If your relative has difficulty using the telephone, British Telecom have a useful leaflet giving details of special phones, including models with push buttons and amplifiers.

LEADING AN ACTIVE LIFE

It is very important to try to lead as full and active a life as possible even if you do have to care for someone who is ill or frail or has a disability. If you (or the person you care for) spend a large proportion of the day without physical or mental stimulation this can lead to boredom, frustration and insomnia.

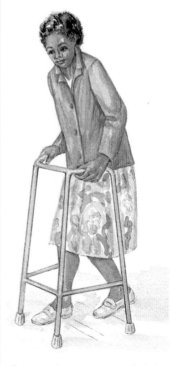

Encourage the person you care for to be independent.

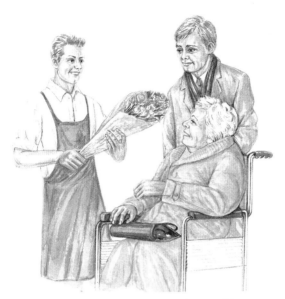

Try to lead as full and active a life as possible.

Although it may be quicker to do something yourself, it is in your own best interests to encourage the person you care for to remain independent. This not only gives them a sense of achievement but means less work for you. If they have problems with manual dexterity, an occupational therapist may be able to advise on adaptations which would make it easier for them to join in household activities.

If your relative is prevented from enjoying hobbies such as television, reading, painting, knitting or sewing, for example, because of sight problems, you might like to contact the Partially Sighted Society who provide large print cards and crosswords. The RNIB run a leisure service which can provide details of games devised and adapted to allow visually impaired people to play. You could also subscribe to the RNIB Talking Book Service or the Talking Newspaper Association of the UK.

Your town hall, local leisure centre and library are all good sources of information about activities in your area. If you or your relative has an interest in a particular hobby, such as sport, fishing or visiting gardens, the relevant organisation will be able to give you advice about disabled access to facilities and venues.

WHEELCHAIRS

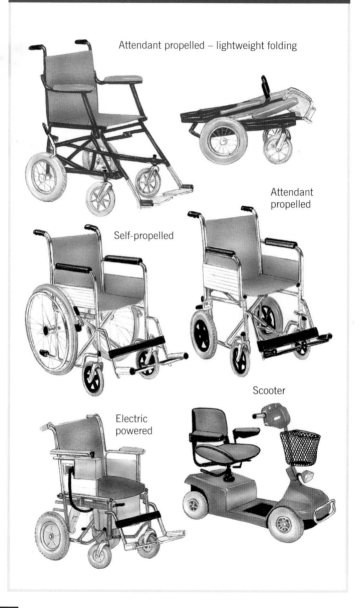

Attendant propelled – lightweight folding

Attendant propelled

Self-propelled

Scooter

Electric powered

MOBILITY

Anything that improves the mobility of the person you are caring for will widen the range of activities you can do and there are many organisations that can help in this respect.

Exercise can help improve mobility and sleep patterns, but consult your doctor first if your relative is unused to physical activity. The Sports Council or your local leisure centre will have information on local amenities that could get you started.

If the person you care for needs a wheelchair for long-term use you will be supplied with one by the NHS. If you want a wheelchair for a short time – perhaps for a holiday or day out – your local Red Cross may be able to lend you one. The chair needs to be matched to the user, taking into account needs and preferences and the environment in which it will be used. An occupational therapist will be able to give you advice on this. If your relative wants a wheelchair that is not available on the NHS you may get help to buy one through a charity such as Motability or the Mobility Trust. Information on racks to carry wheelchairs on cars is obtainable from the Disabled Living Foundation. Many shopping centres now lend wheelchairs for use around the shops for anyone who finds it difficult to walk.

A wheelchair gives the user freedom to move around so that they have more control over their lives. However, it takes time to get used to using a wheelchair and practice is needed to be perfect. Sometimes it may be necessary for the person to adapt their clothes if they spend long periods of time sitting in a wheelchair (see box on page 22).

Many people are put off doing things because of a lack of transport, but there are usually local community transport schemes available, so do ask. If your relative is under 65 years of age and has mobility problems, find out whether they are entitled to the disability living allowance (DLA) mobility component.

Motability is an organisation that can help you to use your DLA mobility money to buy or hire a specially adapted car. If the person you care for qualifies for the highest rate of the DLA mobility component, they can also apply for exemption from road tax. They do not have to drive the vehicle providing it is registered in their name and used on their behalf. The Orange Badge Scheme can be applied for through your local social services department to enable you to park nearer to shops, public buildings, etc. There may be a small charge. You may need advice on where to get aids and equipment.

ADAPTATION OF CLOTHES FOR A WHEELCHAIR

- Garments need to be looser at waist band, hip and crotch
- Trousers need to be cut higher at the back and slightly longer in the leg
- Tight, short or very full skirts may be impractical
- Jackets need to be short or possibly cut away at the back
- Fastenings at the back are best avoided
- Long baggy sleeves may get in the way of wheelchair wheels

An accessible environment and having the right equipment can together provide the key to mobility and independence for your relative. Some equipment is very complex and expensive, other items may be cheap, simple and very effective to use, but either can make all the difference.

The British Standards Institution sets standards for the construction, installation and use of many items of equipment. Be sure the equipment you use bears their 'Kitemark' and the relevant BS number for safety. A word of warning – be careful about buying equipment as it may be obtainable through your social services department or health authority. Check before you spend any money

and get as much advice as you can when choosing.

HOLIDAYS

It is important to try to have holidays if possible to 'recharge your batteries'. There are many holiday centres that will take you both or provide sufficient support so that your relative can go alone. Some schemes offer financial assistance.

Holidays in the British Isles: A Guide for Disabled People, available from RADAR, is an annual guide to accommodation and facilities in the UK. The Holiday Care Service provides a free information service which aims to help people with disabilities and others with special needs to find the right holiday.

KEY POINTS

✓ Ensure your home is safe, pleasant and convenient for both you and your relative

✓ Homes are potentially very dangerous places

✓ Accidents can have very serious implications for sick and elderly people

✓ It is very important that the person you care for tries to lead as full and active a life as possible

✓ Try to encourage the person you care for to retain some independence

✓ Improving mobility will widen the range of activities of the person you care for

Safer moving and handling

You may often have to help the person you care for to move around. It is important you do this for them but especially important that you do it the right way. Lifting and moving weights the wrong way can damage your back or give rise to other physical problems. Your district nurse or physiotherapist should be able to advise you about the best ways for moving and handling. It is preferable to use moving and handling equipment for safety.

GOLDEN RULES FOR MOVING AND HANDLING

- Always keep your back straight. Bend at the knees and/or hips instead. This way you can keep your back straight even when bending over a bed.

- Make your stomach and thigh muscles work. Tightening stomach muscles when moving a person from a chair or bed is important for avoiding back strain. To lift from the floor you need to bend your knees, keep the back straight and use your stomach and thigh muscles.

- Keep feet apart if lifting heavy awkward weights; a firm base is needed.

- Position yourself close to the person you are helping so that if necessary you can use your body to help them.

- Stand with feet apart when you are about to help to make yourself more stable.

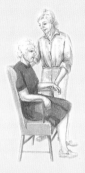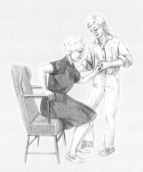

- When you bend or lift, bend your knees and not your back. Many back strains are caused by faulty lifting. Let your legs take the strain.

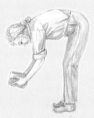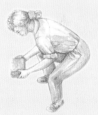

Incorrect   Correct

- Always try to coordinate your actions with the person you are helping. This may not be easy to achieve but can be done with practice. Counting can help to synchronise actions. It may be impossible to complete a move such as standing up from a chair in one action but at each attempt the range of motions becomes greater until the goal is reached.

There is a variety of equipment available from hoists and slings to transfer boards.

The safest method for moving and handling the person you care for is to let them do as much as possible for themselves; try not to lift at all. If you want more comprehensive information about moving and handling many local areas do run moving and handling courses for carers. Contact your local disability information service for details.

STANDING UP FROM A CHAIR

You may solve this problem by raising the height of the seat or putting an extra firm cushion on the seat or raising the whole chair on wooden blocks. Care must be taken, whichever method is used, that the chair is stable. Alternatively you could buy a high chair. Try the following sequence of instructions to get the person you care for to stand up.

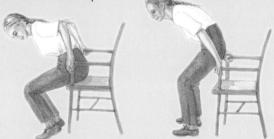

- Move to the edge of the chair
- Place feet on floor well underneath you
- Put feet 8–10 inches apart
- Put hands on the arm of the chair or on the sides of the chair seat
- Now lean forward as far as you can from the hips
- Press down on feet and push forwards with your arms and stand up
- If you cannot stand at first attempt try a rocking motion until the process is achieved

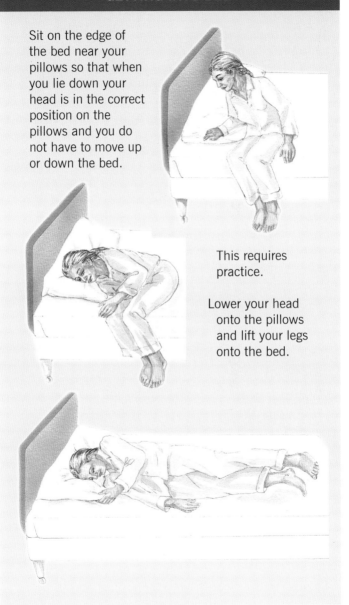

Sit on the edge of the bed near your pillows so that when you lie down your head is in the correct position on the pillows and you do not have to move up or down the bed.

This requires practice.

Lower your head onto the pillows and lift your legs onto the bed.

This is a common difficulty and may be easier to undertake on a firm mattress. If the mattress is too soft place a board under the mattress to support it. To roll over onto the right side, follow the instructions.

- Bend your knees and put your feet flat on the bed. Swing knees to the right side.

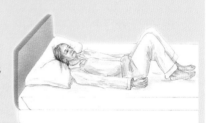

- Grip your hands and lift them up straightening your elbows as you do so.

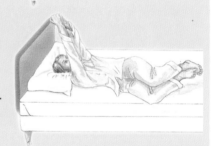

- Turn your head and swing your arms to the right. You may need to repeat this step several times until you have rolled over sufficiently to grip the edge of

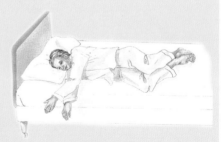

the mattress to pull yourself over further if necessary. Adjust your position until you are comfortable.

Reverse the directions to move onto the left side.

- Lie on your back and put your arms by your side.

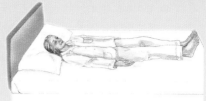

- Lift your head, tuck your chin on your chest and sit up so that you are supported on your elbows.

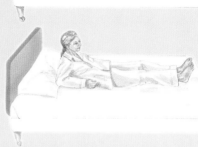

- Keep your head in the same position and sit up taking care to lean well forwards at your hips and support yourself with your arms behind you.

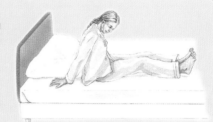

- Move your legs towards the edge of the bed. It may help to count 'one' as you move one leg towards the edge of the bed and 'two' as you move the other leg up to it. Continue as before until you are sitting over the edge of the bed.

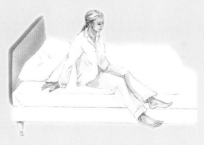

KEY POINTS

✓ Lifting and moving the right way will prevent unnecessary injury

✓ Follow these golden rules when lifting or moving:
  – always keep your back straight
  – bend at the knees
  – keep your feet apart to give stability

Health concerns

There are some health problems which people who lead a largely inactive life are particularly prone to suffer from.

PRESSURE SORES

Pressure sores are likely to occur if either the person has lost sensation in that part of their body from a stroke or other nervous disease or the person has lost the ability to turn over in bed or change position in a chair.

Anyone who has to stay for even short periods in a bed, chair or wheelchair could get a pressure

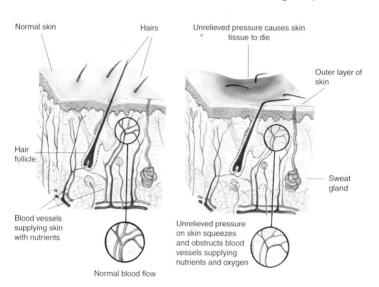

Normal skin

Hairs

Unrelieved pressure causes skin tissue to die

Outer layer of skin

Hair follicle

Sweat gland

Blood vessels supplying skin with nutrients

Normal blood flow

Unrelieved pressure on skin squeezes and obstructs blood vessels supplying nutrients and oxygen

How a pressure sore forms.

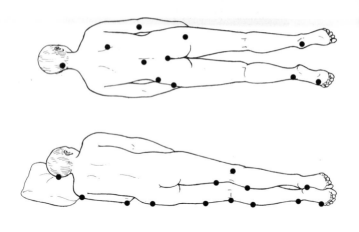

Common sites where pressure sores can develop.

sore. Unrelieved pressure on the skin squeezes and obstructs the tiny blood vessels which supply it with nutrients and oxygen. If the skin is starved for too long the skin tissue dies and a pressure sore forms.

Pressure sores can be very painful and healing may take months and can slow down a person's recovery from other health problems. Areas of skin particularly prone to pressure sores are those that cover a bone on which we sit or lie. When someone has to stay in bed, most pressure sores form on the lower back, the hip bone and the heels.

For those who are confined to chairs, the precise spot where the sore forms depends on how the person sits. Sores can also form between the knees and on ankles, shoulder blades, spine and the back of the head.

Common sites where pressure sores can develop.

PRESSURE SORES

- Someone who is confined to bed can get a pressure sore after as little as one or two hours, and it may happen even more quickly in a chair because the force exerted on the skin is greater.

- Anyone who is not eating a balanced diet and so is not properly nourished may be more susceptible because their skin is less healthy.

- Moisture, including perspiration, will irritate the skin, so pressure sores are more likely in someone who is incontinent of either urine or faeces.

- Both the obese and the very thin person are at increased risk, and tight clothes can contribute to sore formation.

- Individuals who are despondent, confused or generally poorly motivated will be less inclined to move themselves and so more at risk of pressure sores.

- The risk of getting pressure sores is higher if the person cannot move by themselves.

- Moving in the wrong way can add to the risks because shearing forces, which occur when the body tissues are pulled sideways or in opposite directions, can also cause sore formation. This often happens when someone is lifted badly or dragged across the bed.

Pressure sores are potentially very serious, so prevention is better than cure. It's worth taking time to check your relative's skin every morning and evening for any early signs, such as reddened areas that have remained after the position has been changed.

In later stages, the area will be raised, hot and bumpy and will not pale when pressed with a finger. Irregular shallow skin breakdown follows, with blue or black discoloration, and in the final stages deep ulceration, involving fat, muscle and possibly bone.

- Change any wet bedding immediately and, if the skin should be soiled, clean and dry it as soon as possible using a soft cloth or sponge, mild soap and warm rather than hot water.
- Relieve pressure by regular turning or change of position. In bed this needs to be done at least every two hours and twice as often in a chair.
- Make sure that bedding is free from creases or crumbs that can cause friction.
- Avoid massaging the skin.
- Beware of hot water bottles that can burn skin.
- Use a pillow or sheepskin to prevent friction and protect bony areas – between the knees, for example.
- Watch out for tight clothing, studs and buttons on skirts and trousers.
- Keep nails well trimmed to prevent scratching.
- If skin does break contact your district nurse or GP immediately.
- Ask your district nurse or Disabled Living Foundation centre for advice about special mattresses and pillows which relieve pressure in vulnerable areas.
- Try to ensure that your relative has a well-balanced diet.

BLADDER AND BOWEL PROBLEMS

It can be very embarrassing and difficult to discuss the fact that the person you care for has bladder or bowel problems. Often carers just put up with the problems that incontinence brings and never get any proper help. However, there is a great deal of help and advice available for dealing with incontinence; sometimes it can be cured completely and in almost every case there are ways of managing the symptoms. The first priority is to find out the cause of the incontinence. The many causes include urinary infections, loss of muscle tone resulting in stress incontinence, loss of control of the bladder after a stroke, or simply physical difficulties with mobility or dexterity where getting to the toilet or undressing in time is the real problem. Your GP will examine your relative and take a urine sample, and will be able to refer your relative to a specialist doctor or a continence adviser if necessary. The Continence Foundation Helpline is a good starting point for general advice and information. Once the cause of the problem is known, then appropriate action can be taken.

Stress incontinence, where leakage occurs with exertion, for example, coughing or sneezing, can be helped by losing weight, stopping smoking and doing pelvic floor exercises in some cases. Bladder infections may require treatment with antibiotics. Dietary changes may be helpful; reducing or cutting out caffeine and some types of alcohol may help incontinence, although it is important not to cut down on other types of fluid intake too much.

Constipation can be helped by drinking enough fluid and including as much fibre, fruit, vegetables and wholemeal bread in the diet as possible. Laxatives may be helpful but it is not a good idea to use them for long periods unless advised to do so by your GP.

If your relative has physical disabilities or limitations, actually using the toilet may be the difficulty. Distance from or ease of access to the toilet can pose a problem so it is worth thinking about how you can minimise the difficulties.

• **Height:** If the toilet is too low a raised seat may be useful. It is important to make sure you get a

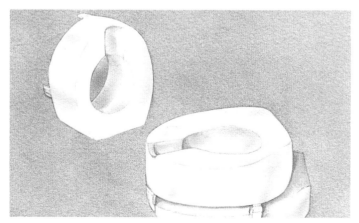

A raised toilet seat may be useful.

seat that clips securely to the toilet bowl for safety.

• **Rails:** A wide variety of rails and frames is available to make independent use of the toilet easier. They can be fixed to the wall or floor and enable the individuals to lower themselves onto the toilet or pull themselves up.

You can get advice on toilet seats and rails from an occupational therapist. Avoid using towel rails or toilet paper holders as supports because these are usually not secure enough.

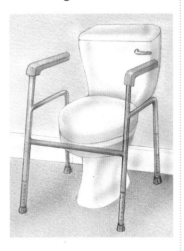

• **Clothing:** It is much easier to remove clothing if it is loose and has as few fastenings and layers to remove as possible. Button fly openings and zips can be difficult to undo but adding a tab to zips or Velcro-fastening fly openings may

help. Boxer shorts or French knickers are easier and quicker to pull down than more close-fitting undies.

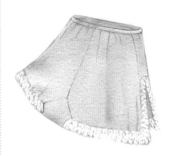

• **Alternative toilets:** If access to the toilet is a real problem it may be possible to get a grant to build a new one but not all houses are suitable. Your social worker could advise on this. A commode may be the answer. This can be discretely curtained off and many commodes now look like normal furniture. Your district nurse could help you get one or the Red Cross may loan one to you. For men, using a bottle (or urinal) may be beneficial and non-spill adapters can be obtained. There are also discrete female urinals available.

If it is impossible to prevent the incontinence there are many different products that can help to manage it more easily and effectively.

• **Pads and pants:** There is a huge

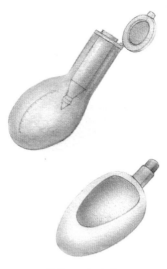

Bottles and urinals.

those who need them, pads can usually be obtained free on the NHS through their district nurse. In some areas, however, people with mild problems may have to buy their pads and those with severe problems may have to supplement the NHS supply.

• **Bed protection:** Absorbent sheets and covers for beds and chairs, some of which can be supplied free by district nurses.

• **Appliances for men:** Some men who have incontinence problems may prefer to use a sheath appliance rather than a pad. These fit over the penis and collect urine into a bag worn on the leg. They are available with a prescription from your GP.

variety available designed to cope with mild to heavy leakage. Most pads are now disposable and held in place with washable pants. For

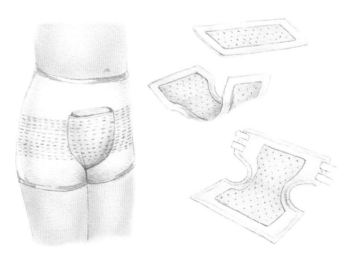

Pads and pants.

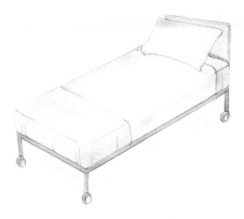

Mattress protection is essential for the incontinent person.

• **Catheters:** Sometimes, a catheter may be inserted to drain urine from the bladder into a bag fitted to the leg. Catheters can also be used intermittently to empty the bladder and these help people who have

INSOMNIA: GUIDELINES

- Diuretics (water tablets) should be taken as early as possible after getting up in the morning
- Constipation may make older people restless and confused, particularly at night; it can also disturb the bladder by increasing the desire to pass urine or by making it more difficult for the bladder to empty
- Late-night drinks should be avoided if visits to the toilet are a problem; check that your relative visits the toilet before going to bed
- Caffeine, alcohol and exercise should be avoided in the evening
- Daytime naps should be avoided if possible
- Going to bed at the same time every night will help your relative to get into a pattern
- Ensure that the bedroom is a comfortable temperature

not been able to find any other way of coping successfully with incontinence.

• **Laundry services:** Some local councils run laundry services.

• **Financial support:** If your relative is receiving income support and needs help to buy a washing machine or extra clothing, he or she can apply for a community care grant from the social fund. You can get details from your local Benefits Agency office.

INSOMNIA

There may be several different causes for insomnia, some of them linked to incontinence. The guidelines in the box on page 38 may help to ease the problem.

Physical pain or discomfort may interfere with sleep. First you need to see if anything can be done to alleviate the pain/discomfort. Your GP may be able to prescribe medication to help the pain from arthritis; pressure-relieving aids such as special mattresses may also be useful.

KEY POINTS

✓ Inactivity can make people more susceptible to certain health problems

✓ Anyone who is confined to bed for even short periods could develop a pressure sore

✓ Check your relative's skin every morning and evening for early signs of pressure sores

✓ Ensure your relative changes position frequently

✓ Dealing with incontinence can be made easier with advice and the right equipment

Illness and ageing

It is impossible to cover all the problems you might come across in your caring role, because each disease or disorder that you may be dealing with will have its own particular features. If your relative does have a specific condition, it will be useful for you to contact the relevant charity or patient association. They often produce very useful literature on coping with particular illnesses. You do not have to join any of the organisations or attend meetings, although many people do benefit from meeting others who care for relatives with similar problems. Some organisations also provide financial support, holidays and friendly visitors. Some more common conditions and problems are looked at below.

DEMENTIA

If your relative has dementia you may experience particular problems with caring. Many people with this condition have periods of agitation if they become afraid or are insecure. What they express at the time may be quite trivial or irrational and may not be the actual cause of their agitation. For example, they may have lost something, or may want to see someone who has been dead for a long time. Repetitive questions are also another aspect of dementia that can be tiresome for carers. In both cases, try to find out what their underlying anxiety is and address that rather than the agitation itself.

Reminiscence therapy is very useful, and simply means talking about events from the past and getting your relative to tell you about their relationship with the particular person they are concerned about. Physical factors such as tiredness, toileting needs, or thirst and hunger can sometimes be the cause of agitation. Boredom may be a source of irritation so try to occupy your relative if possible. The Alzheimer's Disease Society can provide a great deal of advice and support to people caring for all forms of dementia. It also has local groups to support carers.

MENTAL ILLNESS

There has always been stigma around mental illness but with about one in ten people experiencing some form of it at some time, it is much more common than you may have imagined. The government policy of 'care in the community' means that many more people with mental illness are now being cared for at home, and many of their carers may feel frightened and isolated. As with a physical condition, it will help to find out as much as you can and again there are many organisations offering information and advice. If your relative becomes seriously ill the Mental Health Act can be used to take them into hospital, but if at all possible it is preferable to treat someone at home.

OLDER PEOPLE

Almost a quarter of the adult population today is over pensionable age. Do what you can to ensure that your older relative

DEALING WITH SOMEONE WITH MENTAL ILLNESS

- Always try to ensure that your relative takes their prescribed medication. If you have problems encourage them to go back to their GP or community psychiatric nurse.
- A calm and relaxed environment is very important, so do what you can to prevent your relative becoming stressed and angry.
- Be available to provide reassurance and support. Mental illness can be alarming for the person who has it.
- Do take threats of suicide seriously. Contact your GP or community psychiatric nurse.
- Use the national organisations and carers' groups to help you to cope yourself. It is very important that you have support too.

keeps well. This means eating a sensible diet, keeping warm and seeking advice for any minor problems before they get out of hand. Encourage and help them to lead an independent life for as long as possible. If you feel you have tried everything and are still finding it difficult to cope, this does not mean that you have failed. Rather it may mean that you have to reassess your situation and possibly consider residential care for your relative.

MEDICINES

The person you care for may have to take a number of different medicines. Whenever any medication is prescribed for your relative, try to find out as much as possible about the medicine from your GP or pharmacist.

You should make sure the doctor knows about any other medicines that your relative takes, including non-prescription medicines such as simple painkillers or laxatives. It is important to complete courses of medication and could be harmful to stop suddenly, so don't stop your relative taking any prescribed medication without consulting your GP, even if they feel better or have side effects. It can be a worry ensuring that the correct dose is taken at the correct time. Making a chart can help ensure that this is done, or it may be helpful to put out pills for a day or week at a time in special pill boxes to remind you. Your pharmacist may be able to advise on specially prepared medication dispensers you can use.

If the person you care for can manage their own medication, encourage them to do so. If

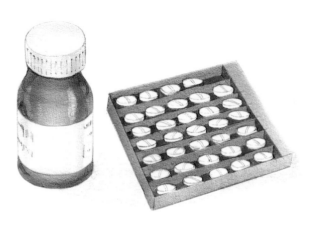

A medicine dispenser is a good idea.

INFORMATION YOU WILL NEED ABOUT MEDICINES

- How often and in what dose must the medication be taken?
- How long should it be taken for?
- When should the doctor be consulted, either because symptoms persist or the next medication review is due?
- Are there any special precautions or warnings that should be followed?
- Are there any side effects or could the medication interact with other medicines? Will side effects wear off, or do they just have to be tolerated? Is there anything that could be done about them?
- Should the medicine be stored in any special way?
- Might the medicine cause any problems when combined with alcohol or certain foods?

opening child-proof medication bottles or blister packs is a problem your pharmacist will be able to offer alternatives. On the other hand, medicines can be very dangerous to confused people, so, if this is the case, make sure you keep all medicines in a safe place, preferably locked away.

Prescriptions can be expensive. Your relative may fit the exemption criteria for free prescriptions, or it may be cheaper to obtain a pre-payment certificate for prescription charges if regular medication is required. Ask your pharmacist. Many offer a prescription collection and delivery service if this is a problem for you.

PALLIATIVE CARE

Palliative care means an easing and controlling of symptoms and may be needed by anyone who has a chronic or malignant disease. Long-term illness or disease can cause considerable psychological and emotional distress, but much can be done to alleviate this distress and help the person to adjust and make the most of their coping skills.

When you are caring for someone in this situation, you may see any one of a number of emotional responses to their long-term illness.

- **Fear:** of increasing dependency, becoming a burden and of the unknown; fear of the progression of the illness and dying.

- **Denial:** which is a coping mechanism used by some people to enable them to live with the illness and its implications.

- **Anger:** which can cause the person you care for to be difficult and abusive, and to refuse your help.

- **Depression:** which should be distinguished from the natural sadness that people feel when they are aware that they can no longer realise their life expectations.

The physical responses to illness may also bring with it practical problems with coping. However, much can be done to prevent, overcome or successfully manage many of the symptoms experienced in illness, and to maintain independence for as long as possible.

Seek and accept help and advice from the many sources from which it is available, and try to think as positively as you can.

TERMINAL CARE

There will come a time when your relative can no longer be treated. Even if you have been expecting this, it may come as a shock to you. If the person you are caring for wants to talk about dying it is important to do this, even if you don't find it easy. Your GP, district nurse, hospice or Macmillan nurse will be able to help you with this. Your own feelings of inadequacy, sadness, fear and anger are to be expected.

The person you care for may also experience wide ranges of emotion. This too is only natural. Caring for someone who is dying at home can be very demanding. Some people wish to die at home; others may feel more comfortable in a hospice with specially trained staff. You can find out what terminal care is available in your area by asking your GP, community nurse or the Hospice Information Service.

When someone is close to death, they may not be responding, but they will still appreciate being quietly spoken to and touched. Hearing is the last sense to go. Remember your words will be heard even though your relative may not be able to respond.

WHEN CARING ENDS

Try not to panic. Death always comes as a shock and you may need to give yourself a little time to calm down before calling for the doctor. He or she will come to confirm the death, and you should then contact the funeral director. All funeral directors offer a 24-hour service and will help you with all the arrangements. You may also want to contact your vicar, priest, church leader or religious leader. The DSS leaflet *What to do After a Death* explains all the practical arrangements necessary. It is not morbid to get this leaflet in advance; it may help you to understand what will be necessary and put your mind at rest.

Both distress and relief are understandable after the death of the person you have cared for. It may help to talk through your feelings with someone close to you: a friend, your GP, a nurse or your religious leader. No two people will react in exactly the same way to a bereavement. You may feel devastated and it can be hard to imagine that you will ever feel any better. You will find, however, that even the worst feelings of despair don't last forever and one day you will be able to think of your relative and remember the happy times that you shared rather than the pain of their death. On the other hand, many people feel relieved when their relative dies. This may be because the person they loved is now free from pain or that their caring role has ended.

For those who would like contact with others in a similar situation, there are local groups in most areas. The organisation Cruse runs social groups where bereaved people can meet others for social contact and mutual support and they can often refer you on to specialist services where necessary. The Lesbian and Gay Bereavement Project offers support to people who have lost a same-sex partner. If you have practical problems to deal with, such as probate or paying for funeral costs, you might want to talk to someone at a Citizens Advice Bureau.

However your caring ends, you are likely to share some experiences with others in similar situations, such as a sense of loneliness. While you were caring for your relative there was always someone around, someone to talk to, even if it was difficult to communicate. You had a role and a purpose and some structure to your day. Now that your caring is over you will need to find new ways to fill your days. It can help to think of a plan in advance and maybe write it down. Decide when you will get up and what you will do and in what order. Occupying yourself will become easier as time passes and, eventually, you will probably wonder how to fit everything in. Make sure you treat yourself regularly too: perhaps an outing to a place you have always wanted to visit or just an afternoon in front of an old film on television.

KEY POINTS

✓ Charities and patient associations can provide useful information

✓ Try to ensure your relative takes their prescribed medication

✓ Seek advice early for any minor problems, before they get out of hand

✓ Make sure your doctor or pharmacist is aware of any medicines your relative is taking before starting any new medication

Caring for yourself

aring can be exhausting, both physically and mentally, and it is important that you look after your own needs as well as those of your relative. This is not selfish; if you neglect yourself physically and become ill or injure yourself, or if you neglect yourself emotionally and become depressed and overtired, the care of your relative will suffer, and the quality of your own life will worsen. Be realistic too about how much you can do; there is nothing to be ashamed of in recognising your limitations and admitting that you are struggling.

LOOKING AFTER YOURSELF PHYSICALLY

Caring is often extremely tiring. As well as being physically hard work, your sleep may be disturbed, or you may sleep very lightly so you wake up in the morning unrefreshed. As a result, you may feel irritable or depressed. When you're exhausted, you can easily find yourself overwhelmed by difficulties that you would normally sail through and you may sometimes feel you simply cannot cope.

A change of routine may help. When broken nights are your problem, you might be able to follow the advice to new parents and take a nap whenever the opportunity arises. Would it be possible to rearrange your sleeping pattern to fit in more with that of your relative? If they have a sleep during the day, maybe you can too. Or is there anything you could do to help your relative to sleep better? (See the section on insomnia on pages 38–9.)

You may suffer from insomnia yourself simply because caring is a stressful occupation. You may lie awake worrying, or be unable to get

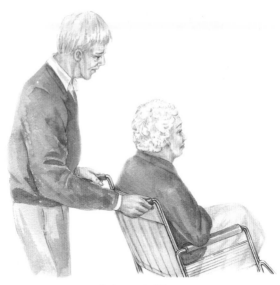

Caring can be tiring.

back to sleep once you've been disturbed. Your GP may be able to help, or you could try relaxation techniques. There may be classes locally, or look in your library for books and tapes on relaxation. A simple but effective technique is as follows: close your eyes for a few minutes and breathe slowly and deeply, then let yourself relax and go as loose as you can when you breathe out. Make time to wind down in the evening before bed; a warm bath, reading a book and listening to music are all relaxing.

Another aspect of looking after yourself physically is making sure that you don't injure yourself. You may often have to help the person you care for to move around and it is important that you do it the right way, otherwise you could well damage your back or create other physical problems. (See 'Safer moving and handling' on page 24 for advice.)

LOOKING AFTER YOURSELF EMOTIONALLY

You may experience a whole range of emotions in connection with being a carer, some of which may feel quite disturbing. Recognising how you are feeling is the first step to dealing with the emotions positively.

Depression

We all have times when we feel down and simply can't handle

everything that life is throwing at us. Usually these feelings go away by themselves after a while, but actual depression is much more serious and can last a long time. It can be hard to admit that you are suffering from it – you may feel that you do not have the right to feel good about yourself.

Once you have acknowledged how you are feeling, the next step is to find someone you trust and can confide in about the way you feel. Don't hesitate to see your GP and tell her or him what is wrong: you will not be dismissed as a time-waster or told to pull yourself together. Doctors are well aware of the problems caused by depression and recognise it as a genuine condition that needs and deserves to be treated. There are various ways of doing this, but there is every chance that you will start to feel a whole lot better once you start receiving the right kind of help.

Guilt

You may have felt pushed into caring for your relative when you don't actually want to or, if you are willing, you may worry that you aren't doing enough or not making a very good job of it. You might end up feeling guilty because you spend so much time on your caring role that there isn't enough left over to devote to other family or friends. If you know or suspect that one day your relative may have to go into a residential care home, you may feel guilty about that too. It's important to admit your feelings to yourself and discuss them with someone if you can. An objective but sympathetic listener will help you to see that your feelings are very natural and help you put them into perspective.

Frustration and anger

It would be surprising if you didn't feel angry or frustrated from time to time and it's unwise to bottle these feelings up. Doing so will make you more stressed and the time may come when you can no longer hide these feelings and just explode. Find safe ways of letting your anger out: walk away from the situation before it becomes a row; once out of earshot you can shout or even punch a pillow and so take out your anger and frustration on inanimate objects; try to relax by deep breathing or using other relaxation techniques; give yourself a few moments alone if you can, and switch off from your worries and immediate concerns. When there is a little more time to spare, perhaps you can take the opportunity to do something that you enjoy as a way of relaxing a little, even if it's just watching a favourite soap on television or reading a chapter or two of your book.

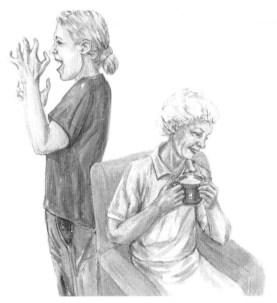

It would be surprising if you didn't feel frustrated or angry from time to time.

Loneliness

Although you may be with your relative for most of the day, you can still feel lonely and isolated. This is even more likely if your relative is confused and does not recognise you, or cannot hold a proper conversation.

You may not have the time to get out and about and meet people as much as you might like or as you used to do. Could your friends come to you even though it is difficult for you to get out? Other options such as arranging a sitter so you can get out more, or joining a carers' support group, are discussed further below.

Stress

Anyone who is caring for a relative with a long-term illness and who has had to make a lot of changes in the way they live is likely to experience high levels of stress. You may develop symptoms such as loss of sleep, headaches, panicky feelings and so on; this is your body warning you that the stress is becoming too much and you need to do something about it. Carers often say that they cannot slow down because the person they care for depends on them; however, pushing yourself too hard is likely to be counterproductive. Think about which parts of your life you find particularly stressful and why. Then think what you would say to another carer if they asked for your advice on that issue. It is often easier to see solutions if you can first distance yourself from your problems. You may then be able to identify some practical steps you can take to improve your situation, or find a new way of looking at things. For example, if you have to learn new skills such as cooking or driving, it helps to see this in a positive light – a chance to extend possibilities rather than an unwelcome necessity.

Sex and relationships

It's very likely that this part of your life will suffer because of your role as a carer, especially when the person you're caring for is someone to whom you're very close emotionally. When that person is your partner, the problems may be even more complex and difficult to tackle. On a very basic level, your caring responsibilities may take so much out of you that you simply don't have the energy to have sex with your partner, or the stress of caring may create tension between you, and you may then feel as if you are letting them down in some way. When the person you are caring for is your partner, you may find that he or she is no longer sexually attractive and your partner might feel the same way about you. Both

caring and being cared for can get in the way of sexual attraction. It may be that you are no longer able to make love in ways that you used to but don't know how to begin discussing this with your partner. Try to be honest about how you feel and encourage your partner to do the same. If either or both of you would like to talk to an outsider, contact an organisation like Relate or the Association to Aid the Sexual and Personal Relationships of People with a Disability.

If the person you have always turned to for love and support is the person you are caring for, many aspects of your previous relationship may now be lost to you. For example, where once you had a relationship of equals you may now have to get used to your partner depending on you to carry out everyday tasks for them. It is vital that you continue to talk to each other as much as possible; sharing these kinds of concerns usually makes them seem more manageable.

SOMEONE TO TALK TO

Many carers feel that they need someone objective to talk to, whether to help sort out a crisis or as long-term support. While a sympathetic friend may be a great support, you may feel guilty about taking up their time, and it may be more helpful to talk to a trained

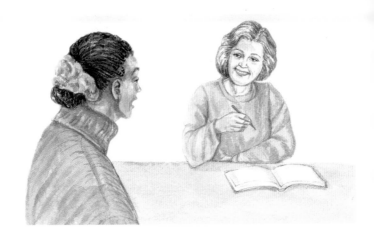

Many carers feel they need someone objective to talk to.

counsellor. You can explore various aspects of your situation and feelings in a way that you cannot usually do with your family and friends, as whatever you say will be private and confidential. Counselling is available from a wide range of sources. You can see a counsellor privately, although it may be expensive, and it is sometimes available on the NHS, so it is worth asking your GP if he or she can refer you. If you wish to talk about a relationship difficulty you may prefer to speak to someone from Relate, who will ask you to pay only what you can afford. If you need someone to speak to urgently, the Samaritans are available 24 hours a day every day. Your Citizens Advice Bureau can tell you what else is available locally.

It might be that you would benefit from joining a group of carers who meet on a regular basis to offer support to one another. It is surprising how much it helps just to know that you are not alone. The Carers National Association will normally be able to give you a contact in your area. You may wish to join the Association as it can help to know that you are part of an organisation that understands how you feel and is trying to make things better for carers. If your relative has a particular condition, check with the relevant organisation to see if they have a support group near you. There are also an increasing number of carers' centres whose staff offer support as well as information and advice to carers. You can find out if there is a centre in your area from the Princess Royal Trust for Carers.

GETTING A BREAK

All of us need a break from time to time and it is not selfish or irresponsible to admit that you simply need a rest. Saying you don't feel you can be on duty all day every day is not saying you don't care. Taking a break may help you care more effectively. On page 60 we look at help you may be able to get from Social Services, but there may also be more informal ways of arranging things.

One way of easing the pressure is to try to reduce the amount you have to get through each day. If you can cut down on household chores for a while, for example, this may

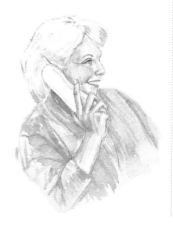

give you a chance to have a much-needed rest. It's also worth considering whether you could ask for more help from other family members. You may feel awkward asking, but sometimes the only reason they haven't offered is because they do not know what to offer, do not like to intrude or simply think that, if you wanted help, you would have said so. Try asking directly; be specific about what you want them to do and when you need them to do it. It may be something as simple as asking them to come and play cards with your mum for the evening while you have a break or something more demanding like having your relative to stay for a few days. If they do not want to help in that way, or are unable to, perhaps they could provide a different kind of help, such as paying for private care for a while. These are all sensitive subjects and only you know whether you can approach your family in this way.

Find out about local sitting services so that you can sometimes go out alone. These may be run by the Social Services/Social Work department but many are run by voluntary groups; try contacting your local volunteer information bureau or Crossroads for more information. Often the local organiser of a carers' group can suggest a way of getting a sitter if this is a problem for you. The Crossroads Care Attendant Scheme has 200 branches all over the country so do see if there is one near you. There may be a waiting list, but don't be put off. Leonard Cheshire has over 40 Care at Home services in the UK providing practical help to people with disabilities and their families. The organisation Community Service Volunteers puts young people who want to do voluntary work in touch with people who need live-in assistance because of a disability.

It is possible to pay for private care at home but this can be very expensive. If you want to use an agency, choose one that is a member of the United Kingdom Home Care Association, which works to a code of practice.

Although using an agency is generally more expensive, at least you don't have to worry about the paperwork and the agency will sort out the workers' tax and National Insurance. You will also be guaranteed alternative staff if the worker is ill or unsatisfactory.

If you choose to recruit a helper yourself you must be careful that you check their references very thoroughly. You will also then be an employer, which means taking on responsibilities such as providing statutory sick pay if the worker is ill, as well as paying tax and National Insurance contributions on their behalf. You may want to get a copy of a booklet called *Recruiting and Employing a Personal Care Worker*, available from the Disablement Income Group.

KEY POINTS

✓ Caring can be exhausting and you must look after your own needs as well as those of your relative

✓ It is normal to feel a wide range of emotions, some of which may seem quite disturbing

✓ It would be surprising if you didn't feel frustrated or angry from time to time

✓ Carers need a break from caring from time to time

The health care system

Caring can be both physically and mentally hard so it is important to have a support system in operation, even if this is only to help you in emergencies, for example, if you are ill. Do not be reluctant to ask for help. Health and Social services are paid for out of your money and everybody has a right to know what and who is available to help. The Patients' Charter sets out the rights to which everyone is entitled in the NHS and sets standards which it should be aiming for. You will be able to get a copy from your GP's surgery.

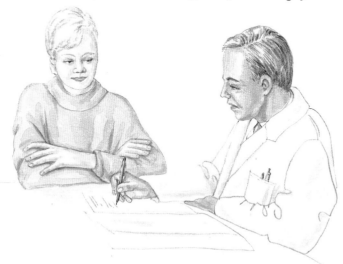

Your GP is the main route to health care and medical services.

YOUR HEALTH CARE TEAM

The main people who will form your health care team are listed below. They also act as 'gatekeepers' to health and social services. They will know what is available in your area and what you are entitled to, and they may also be able to organise these services for you.

Your GP is the main route to health care and medical services. Through him or her you will be able to organise the items in the box.

If you are unhappy with your GP, a simple solution may be to change GP. You can simply go along to a new practice and ask to join. You do not have to give a reason and you do not need the consent of your current doctor. You can obtain a list of local GPs in main post offices, libraries and from Community Health Councils, which will include details such as the gender of the doctor, their qualifications, surgery opening hours and the service provided.

If the problem is more serious, you could consider making a complaint, although it's best to try to resolve the problem with your GP first. A GP who refuses to accept you as a patient does not have to give you a reason but must treat you for up to two weeks while another doctor is found. If this happens you can contact the local Health Authority, who will help you find an alternative doctor. You will find their number in the local phone book. In Scotland contact the Health Board and in Northern Ireland the Health and Social Services Board.

A social worker can help and

YOUR GP IS THE MAIN ROUTE TO THESE HEALTH CARE AND MEDICAL SERVICES

- Referral to a hospital specialist
- District nurse
- Health visitor
- Physiotherapist
- Speech therapist
- Occupational therapist
- Continence adviser
- Wheelchairs
- Places in day hospital or respite care

advise you on a wide range of practical, personal or financial problems. Some areas have specialist social workers who work with older people, or those with sight and hearing difficulties. They can arrange local authority services and put you in contact with local voluntary and self-help groups. Some social workers are attached to GPs' surgeries; otherwise you can contact them through your local social service department (number in 'phone book) by asking for the duty officer. If you cannot leave the person you care for to go and see a social worker they can visit you at home. Social workers can organise services such as:

- Meals on wheels
- Home helps
- Day centres or sheltered work-shops
- Holidays
- Residential care
- Home adaptations and equipment.

District nurses specialise in caring for people in their own homes. They can help you with the practical tasks of caring by undertaking an assessment of need and teaching you how to care, as well as carrying out tasks like care of pressure sores, changing dressings, giving injections and so on. They are also gatekeepers of other nursing and support services such as:

- Night nursing services
- Sitting services
- Continence services
- Equipment loan services
- Chiropody.

Health visitors do not usually undertake practical caring like district nurses, but give health advice. Many health visitors spend most of their time with parents and young children, but some work with elderly people and those with disabilities. They can:

- Help arrange for home adaptations and aids
- Give you day-to-day advice on any problems and concerns you may have.

An occupational therapist can visit you at home and advise on the best type of aids, equipment and adaptations that may be necessary to help you to manage more easily. They may be able to arrange equipment to help you cope with daily living activities such as:

- Eating and drinking aids
- Dressing aids
- Handrails and ramps
- Home adaptations such as a downstairs toilet or shower to assist bathing.

When you visit the GP's surgery you may see the practice nurse, who is responsible for carrying out health checks, giving injections and so on. Some also carry out health assessments for elderly people, run health promotion clinics and may also prescribe medications if they are prescibing nurses.

Community psychiatric nurses specialise in mental illness or caring for people with learning difficulties. They can provide counselling and support for carers as well as for the individual concerned so that he or she can continue to live in the community.

HOSPITAL CARE

In an emergency, your relative is entitled to treatment at any hospital accident and emergency (casualty) department. For all other types of hospital treatment, however, they must be referred by their GP and can't usually choose the hospital they will go to.

You may be worried about how you will cope when your relative comes home if they have been in hospital for treatment. Department of Health guidelines mean that there should be a specific person in the hospital who is responsible for arranging any support and extra care which is needed at home. If you are not automatically given the opportunity to talk to them and be involved in planning for your relative's discharge, ask to see them and make sure any worries you have are attended to properly. If you feel that you are not being offered enough help, don't hesitate to make a fuss and insist that something is done.

Ideally, there should be adequate liaison between hospital and community learning disability nurses and Social Services/Social Work departments to put in place any community care services that are necessary to meet your relative's needs. If your home needs to be adapted in any way before your relative can be discharged from hospital, Social Services/Social Work departments should involve the relevant housing department (Housing Executive in Northern Ireland) as soon as possible. At the very least, a timetable for these improvements should have been worked out before discharge.

You may feel that your relative should not be discharged at all but needs the continuing care of trained professionals within the NHS. Official guidelines specify that the NHS should continue to look after people who have complex medical, nursing or clinical needs, need to have treatments that must be supervised by NHS staff, or are likely to die in the near future. If you feel that your relative still qualifies for NHS care, you can ask for a review of the discharge decision.

MAKING A COMPLAINT

There is one basic difficulty when it comes to complaining about medical treatment which is that it often comes down to a question of individual clinical judgement. There may actually be no such thing as an objectively right or wrong decision about a particular course of action.

However, if you would like to get a second opinion you are entitled to ask for one. Your local Community Health Council can advise you if you experience any difficulty.

If you are considering any further action, it would be wise to discuss it with your Community Health Council or with another organisation such as the Patients' Association before taking things any further. A complaint like this can take a lot of time and energy to pursue and you may want to weigh up the pros and cons carefully, especially if you already have a lot on your plate. This is not to say that you shouldn't go ahead, but rather that you should be fully aware of what you're taking on before you proceed.

KEY POINTS

✓ Health and social services are there to help you

✓ Your GP is the main route to health care and medical services

✓ Social workers can advise you on a wide range of practical, personal or financial problems

✓ District nurses help care for people in their own homes

✓ Health visitors do not usually undertake practical caring, but give health advice

✓ Occupational therapists advise on aids and adaptations to help you manage more easily

Your community care rights

Community care services support people in need of care in the community, and are usually provided by Social Services departments in England and Wales, Social Work departments in Scotland, or the Health and Social Services Trusts in Northern Ireland. These departments must assess anyone who appears to be in need of their help to stay at home, and are also responsible for helping people move to residential care if necessary. You can ask for an assessment, and don't have to be providing care at that time to get one; for example, you may be intending to look after your relative when they come out of hospital. Think carefully about the help you would like and make sure you get your wishes across during the assessment.

An assessment may range from a very simple chat with a social worker to a comprehensive discussion with several professionals, depending on how complex the needs of your relative are. If possible, your relative will participate in the process as well. You also have the right to a separate assessment of your ability to provide, and continue to provide, care, which will be carried out at the same time.

Your assessment must be taken into account when deciding what services are provided to your relative. For example, you may say that you need a regular break in order to help you to carry on caring for your relative. Reassessments should take place regularly, and also if there is a change in your relative's needs or circumstances, or your own.

If the department decides to provide any services, they will write a care plan, explaining the level of services your relative will receive.

As a carer, you have little entitlement to services of your own, although, in practice, almost any care provision you may think of as a service to you is really a service for your relative. For example, respite care (which you may ask for because you need a break) is actually a way of providing care for your relative when it is not convenient or possible for you to do it.

There are a range of other possible services for your relative which may also help you as their carer: a home help, either to shop or to help with personal care; a day centre place, and transport to get there; a meal at home or at a day centre; help to use educational facilities and libraries; adaptations to the home and special equipment; holidays or a telephone. Your relative may still have needs which these services don't meet. The social worker can sometimes then refer your relative to the Independent Living Fund, which may provide regular payments to cover the cost of extra care. The rules are very restrictive, however, for example, the fund cannot help people over 65. Contact the Carers National Association for further advice.

Services that are of major importance to your relative, such as a home care service to help them use the toilet, cannot be reduced or stopped because there is a shortage of money. Charges vary from area to area but Social Services/Social Work departments have to charge what people can reasonably afford. Nobody should be caused hardship or denied access to a service they need because they can't pay. Only the recipient's ability to pay should be considered, not the carer's. If the person can't afford the charge, they can ask for it to be reduced or waived. It will help if they can show that they have a specific difficulty which causes extra expense.

RESPITE CARE

It is sometimes possible to arrange for your relative to stay with a family who are trained and paid by Social Services/Social Work departments. These schemes are usually known as Family Based Respite Care and are arranged through Social Services/Social Work departments. Many schemes now cater for adults as well as for children. The length of stay can vary and it can be an ideal compromise between care at home, which you may feel does not fully meet your relative's needs, and a temporary place in a nursing home, which may be unacceptable to the person concerned.

Residential or nursing home respite care gives you a longer break. It is arranged via the local Social Services/Social Work department, who make the practical arrangements and will help with the fees if your relative has insufficient money to meet them in full. Unfortunately, if the social worker does not agree that respite care is needed, there will be no financial help. They will only pay what they think is reasonable for the type of accommodation, so if they consider a home too expensive, your relative may be asked to go somewhere cheaper, or to pay the difference. If you choose a home in another part of the country, near the sea, for example, they cannot refuse to fund it provided that it is suitable, will take your relative and would cost no more than they would normally pay.

Although it is becoming less common, your relative may be able to go for some respite in hospital. The NHS still has a responsibility for the care of patients with complex medical or clinical needs and for respite health care. NHS care can also be provided in a nursing home. Ask your relative's consultant or GP about this. If you are caring for someone who is terminally ill you could contact the Hospice Information Service to see whether you can get respite care in a local hospice.

RESIDENTIAL CARE

You may have reached the stage when you know you must consider residential care for your relative.

This is a big step which cannot be taken lightly. There are many things to think about and it is important that as far as possible your relative is involved in all of the discussions. Even when you have gone into it all thoroughly and your relative agrees that a home is the best option, you may still find it is hard to let go of your caring responsibilities. It may be that your relative is too confused to make a decision about the particular home that they move into, so you, along with any other concerned family members or friends, will have to choose for them.

Lists of residential and nursing homes can be obtained from the local authority/health authority, from the Health and Social Services Board in Northern Ireland or from the social worker who assessed your relative. The social worker may suggest one or two homes in particular, perhaps where they have placed people before.

Although you should look at these, you might also wish to visit other homes and compare the prices, facilities and attitudes of the staff. Once you have chosen a home, the local authority/ Trust will assess how much, if anything, your relative will have to pay. For more information about finding and paying for residential care for older people, contact Counsel and Care.

How to Complain

At the end of the day, you may be offered fewer services than you need, or inappropriate services, or you may be told that your relative should go into a home, even though neither of you wants this. This sort of dispute does cause much anxiety for carers and those they are caring for. It is up to each local area to decide how much help they will give. This may well mean that you know other people in similar situations who are getting more help than you. Although you may think this is unfair, it is perfectly legal.

If you disagree with the level of services that you have been offered or the charges levied, you do have the right to complain. You can get help with this from an advice centre or one of the organisations supporting people with disabilities. Sometimes your local councillor or MP will intervene on your behalf and this can be effective, so it's worth trying to enlist their backing. The complaints procedure has the following stages.

The informal stage

You have an opportunity to tell the authority what is wrong, and give them a chance to put it right. This is best done in writing.

The formal stage

If the complaint cannot be resolved informally or you choose not to use the informal stage, your complaint must be put in writing to the Designated Complaints Officer, who manages the complaints system. The local authority has 28 days to consider, investigate and respond to the complaint. If it requires more time, it must tell you why and when you can expect a formal decision. In any event, a written decision on your complaint must be provided within three months.

The review stage

Within 28 days of receiving the decision, you can request that the complaint be referred to a review panel, which must be convened within 28 days of receipt of your request. The panel consists of three people, including an independent chairperson. It re-examines the previous decision and must be prepared to listen to both sides and look at any written submissions. Lawyers do not usually attend. Within 24 hours of the hearing, the panel must reach a written decision and forward its recommendations to you and to the authority, which then has 28 days to decide what to do. Within this period it must give you a written decision. Although it is not bound to accept a panel's recommendation, it usually does.

Local Ombudsman procedures

If you are still not satisfied you can

take the matter to the Local Government Ombudsman. Their job is to make sure that local authorities treat people fairly. You must complain within 12 months of the incident or an unsatisfactory conclusion of the complaints procedure.

Compensation may be awarded if you have been treated unfairly.

Court
The only other remedy involves going to court. This can be very expensive and you must seek legal advice if you are considering it. Decisions may be challenged in court by a judicial review.

KEY POINTS

✓ Community care services support people in need of care within the community

✓ Respite care may be arranged to give you a break

✓ Involve your relative as far as possible in the decision over residential care

Money matters

Shortage of money can be a particular problem for carers. When you first start caring, your expenses will probably go up, and if you have to leave work at the same time, it will almost certainly be hard to make ends meet. Make time to work out your financial position in detail: there may be ways you can increase your income or reduce your outgoings. If you find the debts are starting to mount, contact your local advice centre or Citizens Advice Bureau as soon as possible, who will put you in touch with a debt counsellor.

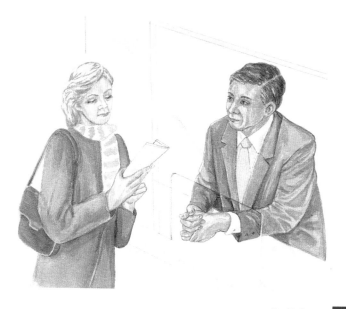

BENEFITS

There may well be social security benefits to which you or your relative are entitled. The rules are often complicated so check out your own situation carefully, and if necessary get advice. You could contact Citizens Advice Bureaux, independent advice centres, welfare rights units, associations for people with disabilities, Age Concern, carers' projects or Carers National Association.

Benefits for carers

Invalid care allowance (ICA) is the main benefit for carers. You might be able to get this if all of the conditions in the box below apply.

You may not get ICA if you are receiving another benefit which 'overlaps' with it, usually incapacity benefit, retirement pension, widow's pension or the jobseekers' allowance. People who are studying more than 21 hours a week cannot get ICA even in the holidays. Only one person can get ICA for each person receiving disability living allowance (DLA) or attendance allowance (AA).

If your relative lives alone (or only with other people who get DLA or AA) and receives income support, housing benefit or council tax benefit/rate rebate, these benefits will include an extra amount called the severe disability premium. This is only paid if they live alone and no one gets ICA for looking after them, so if you claim ICA they will lose this money.

Once you are eligible for ICA, any income support, housing benefit or council tax benefit/rate rebate you get is recalculated under

ELIGIBILITY FOR ICA

- You are at least 16 but under 65 and look after a disabled relative or friend for at least 35 hours a week.

- You do not earn more than £50 a week after expenses.

- The person you look after gets attendance allowance (AA) or the disability living allowance (DLA) care component at the middle or higher rate. These two benefits are explained in more detail later.

the more generous rules for carers, adding in a 'carer premium'. Most carers will get a Class 1 National Insurance Credit for each week ICA is paid. This will make sure that you do not get less state retirement pension because of the years that you have spent caring.

Low income benefits

There may be other benefits that you can get if you or your relative is on a low income. These include income support, housing benefit, council tax benefit/rate rebate, health benefits such as help with dental treatment and glasses, or access to the Social Fund, a system of grants and loans from the Benefits Agency. Get advice if you think you may not be getting all the benefits you are entitled to.

The council tax system has special provisions which may affect carers and those they care for. Properties are exempt from council tax if:

- They are left empty because the resident is in hospital or residential care.

- They are left empty because the person is living elsewhere to receive personal care; for example, if your mother moves in with you so you can look after her.

- They are left empty because a carer has gone to live in someone else's home in order to be able to provide care; for example, if you move in with your mother to look after her.

- They are occupied only by people with severe mental impairment; for example, if your father has Alzheimer's disease and lives alone.

You can claim a 25 per cent discount if you live alone. If no one is regarded officially as living in the household the discount is 50 per cent. When counting how many people live in a household, certain people are ignored completely. They are 'invisible', and include:

- People who are severely mentally impaired, for example, those with dementia.

- Live-in care workers provided by a charity, for example, Community Service Volunteers.

- Carers – but only if they are living with and caring for a person with a disability who is not their spouse, opposite sex partner or child under 18. The person being cared for must receive the higher rate of AA or DLA care component and the carer must be providing at least

Incapacity Benefit: Your relative may be eligible for this if:

- They are of working age but are prevented from doing so by illness or disability.
- They have paid sufficient National Insurance contributions. This means that they must have been an employee or self-employed at some point.

Severe Disablement Allowance: This may be appropriate for your relative if:

- They are of working age but have been too sick to work for 28 weeks and they have a severe disability or developed their disability before the age of 20.
- They have never worked or have not worked for some time or didn't earn enough to pay National Insurance. This benefit doesn't depend on National Insurance contributions.

Disability Living Allowance: Your relative might be able to get this if:

- They are aged under 65 with a disability and one of the following:

35 hours a week of care on average.

The disability reduction scheme means that, if one of the rooms in a property is used mainly by the person with a disability, the council tax payer can apply to be charged as if the property was in the band below. You may qualify if a downstairs room is used as a bedroom or if a wheelchair is used inside the property.

OTHER SOURCES OF MONEY
The only tax allowance specially for

- They need help with personal care or someone to watch over them to make sure they are safe. Unless they are terminally ill, this help must have been needed for at least three months. The DLA care component will then be paid at one of three rates – lower, middle or higher.

- They are over the age of 5 and either can hardly walk or need someone to guide them when they are out. The DLA mobility component will then be paid at one of two rates – lower or higher. A person with a disability may get either or both care and mobility components.

Attendance Allowance: Your relative may be eligible if:

- They are over 65 and have a disability.
- They need help with personal care or someone to watch over them to make sure they are safe.

This benefit is like the DLA care component described above except that there are only two rates, higher or lower, and there is no help with mobility needs.

carers is the additional personal tax allowance. This is payable on top of the married couple's tax allowance to married men and women. You must have at least one dependent child and a husband or wife who is unable to look after him- or herself for the whole of the tax year because of illness or disability.

If the person you care for has been disabled in an accident, do seek legal advice as to whether you can get compensation. People on a low income may get legal aid to help with the costs.

Charities and benevolent funds provide valuable help for carers and people with disabilities by giving

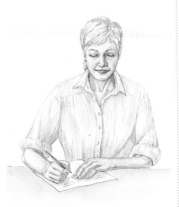

Libraries and advice centres are a useful reference source.

money for essential items. Some give lump sum grants and others weekly allowances. You may be eligible for help because of a link with a job you once had, the particular condition which your relative has, because of where you live or on more general grounds. Libraries and advice centres usually have a book called *A Guide to Grants for Individuals in Need*, listing most of the major funds together with details of whom they can help and how to apply.

DEALING WITH YOUR RELATIVE'S MONEY

- Your relative may be mentally capable but unable to get out.
- If the person's only income is Social Security benefit, you may be able to become their agent. You would always be able to cash their order book. Apply on form AP1, available from the Benefits Agency.
- If they have a bank or building society account you could consider changing this to a joint account.
- Your relative could give you a third party mandate to operate any accounts in their sole name.
- If your relative has very complicated financial affairs, you may have to consider a power of attorney which gives you legal control of someone's money. The power will automatically cease if the person later becomes mentally incapable, unless you make it an enduring power (continuing power in Scotland). You need to think about this now, because after a person becomes incapable, no new powers can be made. You should both seek independent advice before going ahead.

DEALING WITH YOUR RELATIVE'S MONEY

There may be a time when the person you care for can no longer manage their own money. The course of action you should take will depend on their condition and financial circumstances.

If the person you care for is already incapable because of mental disorder, your action will depend on their income. If their sole income is Social Security benefit you could apply, on form AP1, to be their appointee. This means in effect you 'become' them for the purposes of a claim and all correspondence then comes to you.

If the person you care for has another source of income, for example, an occupational pension, your only option, if you do not have enduring power of attorney, is to apply to the Court of Protection if you live in England or Wales (the Office of Care and Protection in Northern Ireland). They exist to look after the affairs of people incapable by reason of mental disorder. They will appoint a receiver (controller in Northern Ireland) to manage the person's affairs. If no one is willing to apply, the receiver/controller can be a solicitor or a bank manager. If the person you care for lives in Scotland, you have to go through a solicitor or accountant who applies to the court to become a 'curator bonis'. This is a costly and difficult procedure and is not recommended except in dealing with very large estates.

KEY POINTS

✓ Shortage of money can be a particular problem for carers

✓ There may well be social security benefits to which you or your relative are entitled

✓ Invalid care allowance (ICA) is the main benefit for carers

✓ There may be other benefits available if you or your relative is on a low income

Useful addresses

Addresses are listed under the following headings:

* Advice
* Ageing
* Benefits
* Bereavement
* Caring
* Counselling
* Disability
* Equipment
* Health services
* Illnesses
* Legal matters
* Mental health
* Residential care
* Volunteers.

ADVICE

Citizens Advice Bureaux
The address of the nearest CAB will be listed in your telephone book.

AGEING

Action on Elder Abuse Response Line
Astral House, 1268 London Road,
London SW16 4ER
Helpline: 0800 731 414
Fax: 0181 679 4074
Email: aea@ace.org.uk

Telephone advice for people concerned about abuse of an elderly relative.

Age Concern England
Freepost (SW30375), Ashburton
Devon TQ13 7ZZ
Tel.: 0800 009966 (7 days; 7 a.m.–7 p.m.)
Web site: www.ace.org.uk

Age Concern Scotland
113 Rose Street, Edinburgh EH2 3DT
Tel.: 0131 220 3345
Fax: 0131 220 2779

Age Concern Northern Ireland
3 Lower Crescent, Belfast BT7 1NR
Helpline: 01232 233323
Tel.: 01232 245729
Email: ageconcern.ni@btinternet.com

Age Concern Cymru
4th Floor, 1 Cathedral Road, Cardiff CF1 9SD
Tel.: 01222 371566
Fax: 01222 399562
Email: accymru@ace.org.uk

Advice and help for older people and their carers. Provide a wide range of factsheets and have local offices all over the country.

Counsel and Care
Twyman House, 16 Bonny Street, London
NW1 9PG
Helpline: 0834 300 7585
Tel.: 0171 485 1550
Fax: 0171 267 6877

Provides advice and information on a wide

variety of subjects relating to people over pensionable age, including residential care.

Elderly Accommodation Counsel
46a Chiswick High Road, London W4 1SZ
Tel.: 0181 995 8320
Fax: 0181 995 7714
Email: enquiries@e-a-c.demon.co.uk

Advice and information on all forms of accommodation for older people, including advice on fees for residential and nursing home care.

Help the Aged
St James Walk, Clerkenwell Green, London EC1R 0BE
Tel.: 0800 650065 (Mon–Fri; 9 a.m.–4 p.m.)

BENEFITS

Benefits Agency
The address of your local Benefits Agency will be listed in your telephone book. Benefits Enquiry Line: England, Scotland and Wales 0800 882200, Northern Ireland 0800 220674.

BEREAVEMENT

Compassionate Friends
53 North Street, Bristol BS3 1EN
Helpline: 01179 539639 (7 days; 9.30 a.m.–10.30 p.m.)

Offers help and support for bereaved parents and their families.

Cruse Bereavement Care
Cruse House, 126 Sheen Road, Richmond, Surrey TW9 1UR
Tel.: 0181 940 4818 (Mon–Fri; 9.30 a.m.–4 p.m.)

Offers both free practical and emotional advice after a bereavement. They have groups all over the country.

Lesbian and Gay Bereavement Project
Vaughan M. Williams Centre, Colindale Hospital, London NW9 5HG
Helpline: 0181 455 8894 (7–12 p.m.)
Web site: www.members.aol.com/LGBP

Support for people who have lost a same-sex partner.

National Association of Bereavement Services
20 Norton Folgate, London E1 6DB
Referral line: 0171 247 1080 (Mon–Fri; 7–12 p.m.)

Directory of bereavement services.

National Association of Widows
54/57 Allison Street, Digbeth, Birmingham B5 5TH
Tel.: 0121 643 8348

They have branches nationwide which provide support to all widows, including a contact list for younger widows. Widowers should contact Cruse or the National Association of Bereavement Services.

CARING

Carers National Association
20–25 Glasshouse Yard, London EC1A 4JT
Helpline: 0345 573369 (Mon–Fri; 10–12 a.m., 2–4 p.m.)
Tel.: 0171 490 8818
Fax: 0171 490 8824
Email: kerry@ukcarers.org.uk
Web site: www.carersuk.demon.co.uk

Information on any aspect of caring. For information about local support and services in Scotland, Wales and Northern Ireland contact the following Carers National Association offices.

Scotland: 3rd Floor, 162 Buchanan Street, Glasgow G1 2LL
Tel.: 0141 333 9495

Fax: 0141 353 3505
Email: internet@carerscotland.demon.co.uk
Wales: Pantglas Industrial Estate, Bedwas,
Newport NP1 8DR
Tel.: 01222 880176
Fax: 01222 886656
Northern Ireland: 3rd Floor, 113 University
Street, Belfast BT7 1HP
Tel.: 01232 439843
Fax: 01232 329299
Email: marie@carersni.demon.co.uk

Crossroads
England: 10 Regent Place, Rugby,
Warwickshire CV21 2PN
Tel.: 01788 573653
Fax: 01788 565498
Email: crossroads.rugby@pipemedia.co.uk
Wales: Ground Floor, Unit 5, Coopers Yard,
Curran Road, Cardiff CF1 5DF
Tel.: 01222 222282
Fax: 01222 238258
Scotland: 24 George Square,
Glasgow G2 1EG
Tel.: 0141 226 3793
Fax: 0141 221 7130
Email: enquiries@crossroads-scot.k-web.com
Northern Ireland: 7 Regent Street,
Newtownards, Co. Down BT23 4AB
Tel.: 01247 814455
Fax: 01247 812112

Provides paid, trained care attendants to go
into the home providing respite care.

Princess Royal Trust for Carers
142 Minories, London EC3N 1LS
Tel.: 0171 480 7788
Fax: 0171 481 4729
Email: PRT4C@aol.com

Provides details of the nearest centre to you
which offers information and support for
carers.

United Kingdom Homecare Association
42B Banstead Road, Carshalton Beeches,
Surrey SM5 3NW
Tel.: 0181 288 1551
Fax: 0181 288 1550

Will give you details of member home care
agencies in your area.

Counselling

British Association for Counselling
1 Regent Place, Rugby,
Warwickshire CV21 2PJ
Tel.: 01788 550899
Fax: 01788 562189
Email: bac@bac.co.uk
Web site: www.counselling.co.uk

Can provide a list of counsellors in your area
on receipt of an A5 SAE. There is a charge of
£1 for any additional areas.

Relate
See your local phone book. Runs local
couple counselling services.

The Samaritans
0345 909090. 24-hour listening ear for
anyone in distress.

Disability

Association to Aid the Sexual and Personal Relationships of People with a Disability (SPOD)
286 Camden Road, London N7 0BJ
Tel.: 0171 607 8851
Fax: 0171 700 0236

Information and advice on sexual and
relationship problems.

Disabled Living Centres Council
1st Floor, Winchester House,
11 Cranmer Road, London SW9 6EJ
Tel.: 0171 820 0567

Fax: 0171 735 0278
Email: dlcc@dlcc.demon.co.uk

Will tell you if there is a Disabled Living Centre near you where disabled people, elderly people and carers can see various types of equipment.

Disabled Living Foundation
380/384 Harrow Road, London W9 2HU
Helpline: 0870 603 9177
Minicom: 0870 603 9176 (Mon–Fri; 10 a.m.–4 p.m.)
Tel.: 0171 289 6111
Fax: 0171 266 2922
Email: dlfinfo@dlf.org.uk
Web site: www.dlf.org.uk

Advice and information about equipment for disability.

Disablement Income Group
Unit 5, Archway Business Centre, 19–23 Wedmore Street, London N19 4RZ
Tel.: 0171 263 3981

Advice on financial matters for disabled people. Produces a useful guide to recruiting and employing a care worker.

Disability Scotland
Princes House, 5 Shandwick Place, Edinburgh EH2 4RG
Tel.: 0131 229 8632
Fax: 0131 229 5168
Email: disability.scotland@virgin.net
Web site: www.dis_scot.gcal.ac.uk

Advice for disabled people in Scotland.

Holiday Care Service
2nd floor, Imperial Buildings, Victoria Road, Horley, Surrey RH6 7PZ
Tel.: 01293 774535
Fax: 01293 784647

Advice on holidays for disadvantaged people, disabled people and carers.

Independent Living Fund
PO Box 183, Nottingham NG8 3RD
Tel.: 0115 942 8191
Fax: 0115 929 3156

Money for severely disabled people to buy in care.

Leonard Cheshire
30 Millbank
London SW1P 4QD
Tel.: 0171 802 8200
Fax: 0171 802 8250
Email: lcf@community.co.uk
Web site: www.leonard-cheshire.org

Care schemes for disabled people.

Mobility Trust
50 High Street, Hungerford, Berks RG17 0NE
Tel.: 01488 686335
Fax: 01488 686336
Email: mobility@mobilitytrust.org.uk

The trust lends disabled people equipment, such as powered wheelchairs.

Motability
Goodman House, Station Approach, Harlow Essex CM20 2ET
Helpline: 01279 635666

Advice and help to buy cars and powered wheelchairs for disabled people on mobility component of Disability Living Allowance.

RADAR
12 City Forum, 250 City Road, London EC1V 8AF
Tel.: 0171 250 3222 (Mon–Fri; 10 a.m.–4 p.m.)
Fax: 0171 250 0212
Email: radar@radar.org.uk
Web site: www.radar.org.uk

Information and advice for disabled people.

Wales Council for the Disabled

Disability Wales, Llys Ifor, Crescent Road, Caerphilly CF83 1XL
Tel.: 01222 887325
Fax: 01222 888702
Email: info@dwac.demon.co.uk

Advice for disabled people in Wales, referral to local groups.

Winged Fellowship

20-32 Pentonville Road, London N1 9XD
Tel.: 0171 833 2594
Fax: 0171 278 0370
Email: wft@wft.org.uk
Web site: www.wft.org.uk

Holidays for disabled people.

EQUIPMENT

DLF – see Disability

Naidex

Reed Exhibition Company-Naidex, Oriel House, 26 The Quadrant, Richmond, Surrey TW9 1DL
Tel.: 0181 910 7873
Fax: 0181 910 7926
Email: michelle.cunningham@reedexpo.co.uk

Organises regular exhibitions of equipment and services for elderly or disabled people.

British Red Cross Society

9 Grosvenor Crescent, London SW1X 7EJ
Tel.: 0171 235 5454
Fax: 0171 245 6315
Email: information@redcross.org.uk
Web site: www.redcross.org.uk

Local branches can loan equipment.

HEALTH SERVICES

Action For Victims of Medical Accidents

44 High Street, Croydon, Surrey CR0 1YB
Tel.: 0181 686 8333
Fax: 0181 667 9065

Advice for people who have suffered as a result of medical treatment or failure to give medical treatment.

The British Society of Dentistry for the Handicapped

Hon. Secretary, Dental Department, Town Centre Clinic, Caradoc Road, Cwmbran, Gwent NP44 1XJ
Tel.: 01633 838356

Community Health Council/Local Health Council

Address in your local phone book. Advice and help with complaints about local health services.

Family Health Services Authority/Health Boards

Addresses and telephone numbers are in your telephone directory or from your Citizens Advice Bureau or library. Gives information about local health services, e.g. doctors and dentists in your area.

Health Service Ombudsman

Investigates complaints about the health service.
England: 11th Floor, Mill Bank Tower, Millbank, London SW1P 4QP
Tel.: 0171 276 2035
Fax: 0171 217 4000
Web site: www.ombudsman.org.uk
Scotland: 28 Thistle Street Edinburgh EH2 1EN
Tel.: 0131 225 7465
Fax: 0131 226 4447
Wales: 5th floor, Capital Tower, Greyfriars Road, Cardiff CF1 3AG

Tel.: 01222 394621
Fax: 01222 226909
Northern Ireland: Office of Northern Ireland Commissioner for Complaints, 33 Wellington Place, Belfast BT1 6HN
Tel.: 01232 233821

Hospice Information Service
St Christopher's Hospice, 51–59 Lawrie Park Road, Sydenham, London SE26 6DZ
Tel.: 0181 778 9252, ext. 262

Local Government Ombudsman
Investigates complaints about local government (Boards in Northern Ireland).
England: 21 Queen Anne's Gate, London SW1H 9BU
Tel.: 0171 915 3210
Fax: 0171 233 0396
or The Oaks, Westwood Way, Westwood Business Park, Coventry CV4 8JB
Tel.: 01203 695999
or Beverley House, 17 Shipton Road, York YO3 6FZ
Tel.: 01904 663200
Scotland: 23 Walker Street, Edinburgh EH3 7HX
Tel.: 0131 225 5300
Fax: 0131 225 9495
Wales: Derwen House, Court Road, Bridgend CF31 1BN
Tel.: 01656 661325
Northern Ireland: The Ombudsman is the same as for the Health Service, see above.

Patients' Association
PO Box 935, Harrow HA1 3XJ
Helpline: 0181 423 8999

Illnesses

Alzheimer's Disease Society
Gordon House, 10 Greencoat Place, London, SW1P 1PH
Helpline: 0845 300 0336
Fax: 0171 306 0808

Email: info@alzheimers.org.uk
Web site: www.alzheimers.org.uk

Information and support for families affected by Alzheimer's disease.

Arthritis Care
18 Stephenson Way, London NW1 2HD
Tel.: 0800 289170

Information, support and holiday centres for people with arthritis.

British Diabetic Association
10 Queen Anne Street, London W1M 0BD
Helpline: 0171 636 6112
Fax: 0171 637 3644
Email: diabetes@diabetes.org.uk
Web site: www.diabetes.org.uk

British Epilepsy Association
40 Hanover Square, Leeds LS3 1BE
Helpline: 0800 309030

Cancerlink
11–21 Northdown Street, London N1 9BW
Tel.: 0800 132905

Support and information on all aspects of cancer.

The Continence Foundation
307 Hatton Square, 16 Baldwin Gardens, London EC1N 7RJ
Helpline: 0171 831 9831
Tel.: 0171 404 6875
Fax: 0171 404 6876
Email: continence.foundation@dial.pipex.com
Web site: dspace.dial.pipex.com/continence.foundation

Has a range of literature for people with continence problems. Callers can speak to nurses with a specialist knowledge of bladder and bowel problems. They also hold a database of service and products throughout the UK.

Incontinence helplines

Bard: 0800 591783 (12.30–4.30 weekdays).
Coloplast Service: 0800 220622 (Mon–Fri;
8 a.m.–7 p.m.)
Hollister Ltd (specialises in ostomy care):
0800 521377.

All helplines have trained advisers who give
confidential information. Those listed above
are run by commercial companies but are
Freephone numbers. See also The
Continence Foundation.

ME Association

Stanhope House, High Street, Stanford Le
Hope, Essex SS17 0HA
Helpline: 01375 361013 (Mon–Fri;
1.30 p.m.–4 p.m.)
Tel.: 01375 642466

Motor Neurone Disease Association

PO Box 246, Northampton NN1 2PR
Helpline: 08457 626262
Fax: 01604 624726

Multiple Sclerosis Society

25 Effie Road, London SW6 1EE
Helpline: 0171 371 8000 (Mon–Fri;
10 a.m.–4 p.m.)
Tel.: 0171 610 7171
Fax: 0171 736 9861
Email: info@mssociety.org.uk
Web site: www.mssociety.org.uk

National Back Pain Association

16 Elm Tree Road, Teddington, Middlesex
TW11 8ST
Tel.: 0181 977 5474
Fax: 0181 943 5318
Email: 101540.1065@compuserve.com

National Schizophrenia Fellowship

Provides information and services for those
with schizophrenia and their carers.
England: 28 Castle Street, Kingston-upon-
Thames, Surrey KT1 1SS

Helpline: 0181 974 6814 (Mon–Fri;
10 a.m.–3 p.m.)
Fax: 0181 547 3862
Email: info@nsf.org.uk
Web site: www.nsf.org.uk
Scotland: NSF (Scotland), 40 Shandwick
Place, Edinburgh EH2 4RT
Tel.: 0131 226 2025
Fax: 0131 225 7552
Wales: Suite C2, William Knox House,
Brittanic Way, Llandarcy, Neath SA10 6EL
Helpline: 01792 813052
Tel.: 01792 816600
Fax: 01792 813056
Northern Ireland: Wyndhurst, Knockbraken,
Health Care Park, Belfast BT8 8BH
Tel.: 01232 402323
Fax: 01232 401616

Parkinson's Disease Society of the UK

215 Vauxhall Bridge Road, London SW1V 1EJ
Helpline: 0171 233 5373
Tel.: 0171 931 8080
Fax: 0171 233 9908

Partially Sighted Society

PO Box 322, Doncaster DN1 2XA
Tel.: 01302 323132
Fax: 01302 368998

Royal National Institute for the Blind

224 Great Portland Street, London W1N 6AA
Helpline: 0345 669999
Tel.: 0171 388 1266
Fax: 0171 388 2034
Web site: www.rnib.org.uk

Royal National Institute for Deaf People

19/23 Featherstone Street,
London EC1Y 8SL
Helpline: 0870 605 0123
Tel.: Voice 0171 296 8000
     Minicom 0171 296 8001

Fax: 0171 296 8199
Email: helpline@rnid.org.uk
Web site: www.rnid.org.uk

Royal Society for Mentally Handicapped Children and Adults (MENCAP)
MENCAP National Centre,
123 Golden Lane, London EC1Y 0RT
Tel.: 0171 454 0454

Support, information and help for people with learning difficulties.

Stroke Association
Stroke House, Whitecross Street,
London EC1Y 8JJ
Helpline: 0845 303 3100
Tel.: 0171 566 0300
Fax: 0171 490 2686

LEGAL MATTERS

Court of Protection
Arranges financial affairs for people who cannot manage their own because of mental disorder.
England and Wales: Public Trust Office, Protection Division, Stewart House, 24 Kingsway, London WC2B 6JX
Helpline: 0171 664 7300
Tel.: 0171 664 7000
Fax: 0171 664 7702
Northern Ireland: Office of Care and Protection, Royal Courts of Justice, Chichester Street, Belfast BT1 3JF
Tel.: 01232 235111
Fax: 01232 313508

MENTAL HEALTH

Mental After Care Association
25 Bedford Square, London WC1B 3HW
Tel.: 0171 436 6194
Fax: 0171 637 1980

Provide services in the community for people with mental health needs and their carers.

MIND
Granta House, 15–19 The Broadway,
Stratford, London E15 4BQ
Helplines – London: 0181 522 1728
                    Other: 0345 660163
Tel.: 0181 519 2122
Fax: 0181 522 1725
Email: contact@mind.org.uk
Web site: www.mind.org.uk

A national organisation for people with any mental illness and their carers. They offer legal advice and have regional and local offices.

Northern Ireland Association for Mental Health
80 University Street, Belfast BT7 1HE
Helpline: 01232 237937
Tel.: 01232 328474
Fax: 01232 234940
Email: niamhbel@aol.com

Offers a range of support and services to people with mental health difficulties living in the community.

SANE
1st Floor, Cityside House, 40 Adler Street,
London E1 1EE
Helpline: 0345 678000 (every day; 2–12 p.m.)
Tel.: 0171 375 1002
Fax: 0171 375 2162
Web site:
www.mkn.co.uk/help/charity/sane/index

Supports people with mental illness and their carers, has a database of other organisations and self-help groups.

Scottish Association for
Mental Health
Cumbrae House, 15 Carlton Court,
Glasgow G5 9JP
Tel.: 0141 568 7000
Fax: 0141 568 7001

Provides information about services in
Scotland and publishes a series of leaflets.

RESIDENTIAL CARE

Relatives Association
5 Tavistock Place, London WC1H 9SN
Tel.: 0171 916 6055
Fax: 0171 916 6093

Practical advice about difficulties
encountered in residential care. Has local
support groups for relatives of those in
homes.

VOLUNTEERS

CSV
(Community Service Volunteers)
237 Pentonville Road, London N1 9NJ
Tel.: 0800 374991
Fax: 0171 837 9318
Email: 106167.2756@compuserve.com

Provides full-time volunteers to help you
look after someone.

Council for Voluntary Service
See your local phone book (may also be
listed as 'Volunteer Bureau'), or ask a library
or advice centre where the nearest one is.
Matches volunteers with organisations and
sometimes individuals needing help.

Index